Scabies and Lice Explained

Causes, Prevention, Treatment, and Remedies All Covered!

Information including symptoms, cure, removal, eggs, home remedies, in pets, natural treatment, life cycle, infestation, race specific, and much more.

By: Frederick Earlstein

Foreword

There are many misconceptions and urban "legends" about lice and scabies. The mere mention of these parasites tends to send people into a frenzy of scratching generated by little more than their own over-active imaginations.

Humans recoil in horror at even the word "lice." The presence of these insects and of the human itch mite that causes scabies, are seen as an indication of disease and poor hygiene. People who suffer through an infestation suffer equally from the attached social stigma.

Even more serious is the mistaken conception that lice and scabies are found only among certain ethnic groups. In truth, lice are found all over the world and are no respecters of race, gender, or social status.

Lice and scabies are opportunistic human parasites, thriving in close quarters and taking advantage of circumstances in which people have only a limited ability to bathe or change into clean clothes. This is why the insects are often seen among nursing home residents, or refugees from natural disaster and war.

The generally held belief is that only body lice spread disease, in particular typhus, but this is actually up for debate.

At the time this theory was posited, prior to the publication of Hans Zinsser's definitive study, *Rats, Lice and History* in

1935, body lice were the most prevalent type of lice affecting man.

Zinsser believed that head lice also carried disease; a fact supported by subsequent research in which lice injected with typhus successfully transmitted the germ to a host.

In modern times, head lice are more prevalent than body lice, as pointed out in a 1978 paper for *Acta Tropica* by F. Weyer.

"We have to remember that the number of persons infected with lice has been steadily increasing for more than 20 years, especially in highly developed countries," Weyer wrote.

"Although these 'lice of affluence' chiefly involve head lice, we have to bear in mind that head lice are also able to become infected with and transmit *R. prowazekii* [the infectious agent of typhus], and *Borrelia recurrentis* [the infectious agent of relapsing fever]."

In the case of scabies, caused by the human itch mite, individuals with a compromised immune system are at an especially high risk of infestation, especially if they are living in an institutional setting. Scabies are, however, also regarded as a nuisance rather than a health threat in and of themselves.

Once removed from the social stigma associated with an infestation, it is relatively simple to address and eradicate

Foreword

both lice and scabies. Anti-lice products are available as over-the-counter preparations, while scabies treatments require a prescription from a doctor.

The greatest threat in terms of overall health is typically the development of secondary skin infections as a consequence of open sores that develop from incessant scratching. Intense itching is the number one symptom in all forms of lice and scabies infestations.

The purpose of this text is to demythologize these parasites and to present — in easily understood language — a narrative of their causes, presentation, diagnosis, and treatment.

In our advanced modern state, humans simply forget that we are but one life form on this planet, and are susceptible to becoming hosts for a range of parasites.

Although admittedly an uncomfortable and distasteful topic, lice and scabies can be effectively managed and are not a cause for either shame or censor.

Foreword

Acknowledgments

I would like to express my gratitude towards my family, friends, and colleagues for their kind co-operation and encouragement which helped me in completion of this book.

My thanks and appreciations go to my colleagues and people who have willingly helped me out with their abilities.

Acknowledgments

Table of Contents

Table of Contents

Table of Contents

Table of Contents

The History of Lice and Other Parasites

Using research conducted with DNA, scientists estimate that the human head louse has existed for 5.6 million years virtually unchanged. Basically, these parasites and their closest relatives are quite good at what they do – feeding on blood, reproducing, and making their hosts utterly miserable.

Head lice and body lice, although virtually indistinguishable to the naked eye, likely split into two forms about 107,000 years ago. When archaeologists excavated a site in northeast Brazil in 2000, a nit was found on a 10,000-year-old strand of human hair – the oldest louse/human connection found to date.

Previously, lice were discovered in matted human hair from a 9,000-year-old skull from the Neolithic Era, and on 5,000-year-old Egyptian mummies. In fact, fine-toothed lice combs were included among the artifacts in the great tombs.

Centuries Old Remedies

Over the centuries, plagued by a variety of parasites, man has come up with a wide range of improbable remedies to relieve their infestations. The Ebers' Papyrus from 1536 BC recommended spitting a mouth full of date meal and water on the skin to drive off lice and fleas.

The History of Lice and Other Parasites

The Chinese in 1200 BC were a little harder hitting in their approach, opting for applications of both toxic mercury and arsenic. Undoubtedly, the lice found these substances deadly, but it's likely their human hosts didn't fare too well over the long term either.

Herodotus, writing in 430 BC claimed that Egyptian priests shaved themselves every other day to keep their bodies free of hair, and thus of lice as well. In 330 BC, Aristotle set forth a theory that lice spontaneously generated from the skin of animals.

He went so far as to divide lice into "wild" and "ordinary" varieties, pointing to the exceptional difficulty of ridding oneself of the wild type. In 350 BC he wrote, "Boys' heads are apt to be lousy, but men's in less degree; and women are more subject to lice than men."

The Greek physician Dioscorides of Anazarbus who tended to the men of Nero's army in 64 AD advocated the use of oil of cedar rubs for lice, which he said would also take care of bed bugs. Pliny the Elder in 77 AD was arguably a little more "out there," writing:

"Nits are destroyed by using dog's fat, eating serpents cooked like eels, or else taking their sloughs (shed skin) in drink."

By 100 AD, the ever-determined Chinese eschewed mercury and arsenic in favor of equally deadly wormwood.

In roughly the same period, however, they also discovered a powder ground from the dried flowers of a species of chrysanthemum made an excellent insecticide. It still does. It's called pyrethrum, and remains a major anti-lice remedy today.

Sometime around 1300, Marco Polo is believed to have brought pyrethrum to Europe, but old remedies die hard. Well into the 1960s, doctors at the Royal Edinburgh Hospital in Scotland were still using arsenic preparations to treat lice infestations.

Advances in Science

It was not until 1864, however, that Louis Pasteur demonstrated that Aristotle's theory of the spontaneous generation of insects, including lice, from flesh was in error.

These and other discoveries relative to parasites in humans were greatly aided by the refinement of magnifying devices including microscopes, as well as improved insight into germ theory.

In 1909, Charles Nicolle discovered the link between the spread of typhus and the presence of body lice. By the end of World War I, troops were using insecticide powders to control the spread of lice in the field, a practice continued in World War II with the use of DDT.

Thanks to the use of DDT, infestations of lice, especially head lice, were not common in the developed world between 1945 and 1975, but then the toxicity of DDT was revealed and its use largely curtailed.

In the years since, lice have shown a stubborn ability to develop resistance to a number of insecticides, but rather than travel in search of deadlier poison, modern medicine now opts for pediculicides (anti lice treatments) that suffocate the adults and newly hatched nymphs over at least two treatments.

This approach, paired with vigorous house cleaning and laundering has proven effective without the need for highly toxic agents that can be absorbed into the skin or breathed into the lungs.

A Long Association

One thing is quite clear, however. Mankind has waged a long and running battle against lice – in fact, against parasites of all sorts.

All of the preparations to eradicate the pests – no matter how deadly or outlandish – have also been recommended as a means to fight fleas, ticks, bed buds, and mites like the one that causes scabies in humans.

Scabies and lice are not new problems for man, and they have not been eliminated in the 21st century. Parasites that have been around for millions of years pretty much know how to survive.

The History of Lice and Other Parasites

Certainly having an infestation of any one of these parasites is uncomfortable, and embarrassing. They can, however, be eradicated with a reasonable course of treatment and removal.

It may not be comforting to know that 10,000 years ago that poor soul in Brazil was itching from a lice infestation, but it does show that in some battles, we humans can't always claim to have the upper hand!

Part I – Understanding Head Lice

There are three types of lice infestations. Each of the parasites feeds on human blood, and all are spread by direct contact. Pets and other animals do not pass lice to human beings.

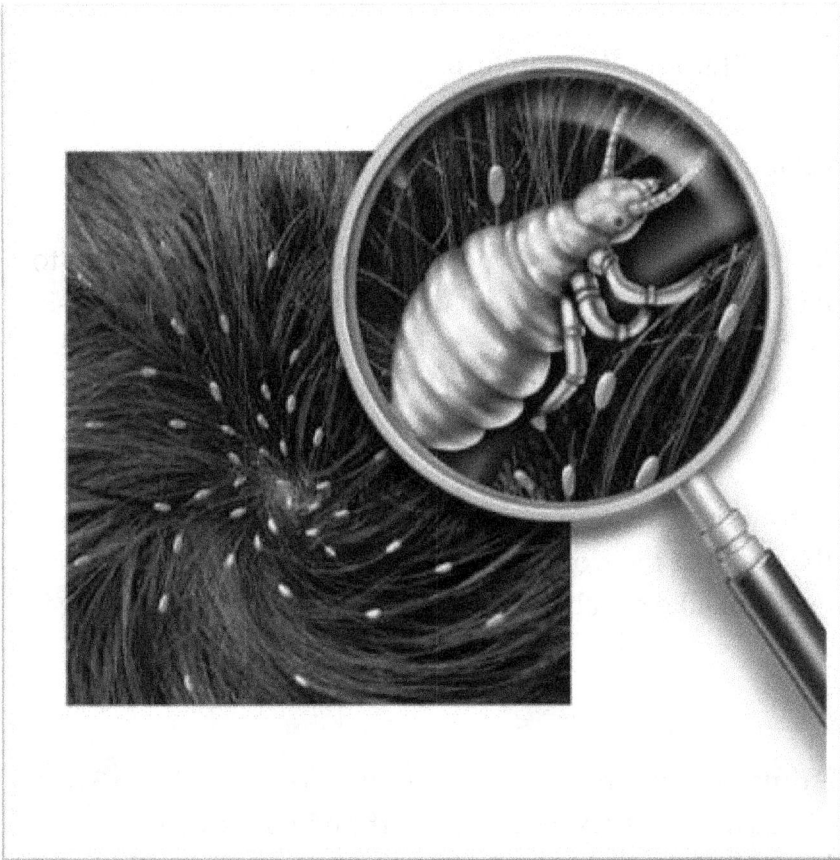

All forms of lice move by crawling. They do not fly or jump. You cannot become infested with lice simply by standing next to or even being in the same room with someone who has the parasites.

If, however, you come into contact with that person, or potentially with something they have worn, transmission is almost guaranteed. The three types are:

- Head Lice (*Pediculus humanus capitis*)
- Body Lice (*Pediculus humanus corporis*)
- Pubic Lice (*Pthirus pubic*)

If a person carries either head or body lice, they are said to have pediculosis. The main difference in these two parasites is that body lice feed twice a day, whereas head lice feed more often. There is also a slight size difference.

If pubic lice are present, the condition is called pthiriasis, or in the common vernacular "crabs." (The name derives from the fact that the front two claws on this species are larger and look like a crab's pinchers.)

Head Lice

Adult head lice reach a length of no more than 2.1 to 3.3 mm. They have six legs, each outfitted with claws or "hooks" at the end used for tightly attaching to the hair shafts where they live.

Part I – Understanding Head Lice

Head lice are found on the head and neck, and occasionally in the eyebrows. Favored spots for high concentrations are:

- the back of the head,
- around the ears,
- and near the neckline.

Adult head lice will deposit their eggs at the base of the hair shaft. The parasites pass through three discernible life stages:

- nit or egg
- nymph
- adult

All three life stages may be present on an infested individual at one time. This is why it is imperative to make sure that all "eggs" have been killed before an individual can be pronounced "clear."

(It's actually a misperception that anti-lice agents kill lice eggs. Most do not. The second treatment is to kill nymphs or juveniles that have hatched since the first treatment.)

Nits or Eggs

The female louse lays her eggs as close to the scalp as possible. The nits become quite firmly attached to the hair shaft, so much so, in fact, that they are very difficult to remove.

Part I – Understanding Head Lice

The eggs that are most likely to hatch in the required 8-9 days are those that have been laid approximately a quarter of an inch (0.64 cm) from the scalp.

Lice eggs will not live more than a week off a human host, and cannot hatch in an environment colder and less humid than the human scalp.

In appearance, the nits are oval shaped and no larger than a knot in a piece of thread. If you were to place a lice egg next to the back of an American one-cent piece, it would fit between the columns of the Lincoln Memorial depicted on the coin.

Nits are yellow or white in coloration, but can sometimes appear to be the same color as the hair of the person on which they are living. The nits are so tiny, it's easy to mistake them for flakes of dandruff or even for drops of hairspray.

Nymph

A nymph hatches from the nit and is an immature form of the adult louse. Their appearance is identical to that of the adult. Nymphs feed on blood and will mature in 9-22 days after hatching.

It is easy to mistake a nymph for an unhatched nit, but generally nymphs are found more than a quarter of an inch (0.64 cm) above the base of the hair shaft.

Part I – Understanding Head Lice

Adult Head Lice

When nymphs have reached full maturity and are classed as adults, they are roughly the same size as a sesame seed. The lice are grey or tan, but may appear darker if they are present in dark hair.

The parasites feed several times a day on blood from the scalp. They can live for 30 days on a host, but will die within 2 days if no host is present.

Adult female lice are capable of laying 6 eggs per day, a fact that perpetuates the infestation and makes eradication more difficult.

This is why anti-lice treatments call for two applications: one to destroy the living lice currently present, and a second to kill those that subsequently hatch.

Distribution and Risk

Lice are distributed globally, and spread most readily among high-risk populations in specific environments. These environments may vary by region and by the degree of development present in the country in question.

In the United States, for instance, head lice are common among groups of children at facilities including, but not limited to:

- child care facilities including day cares

- kindergarten and elementary classrooms
- households with multiple children

Exact figures are difficult to ascertain as head lice can be treated with over-the-counter remedies and are not always reported to health department authorities.

For instance, best estimates suggest that 6-12 million infestations occur annually in the United States among the 3-11 age group.

Over the past few years, cases of head lice have actually increased in the developed world, in part because the parasites have become more resistant to the most common anti-lice agents used in these countries.

Inaccurate Racial Stereotypes

The widely held belief that African-Americans are more prone to infestations of head lice is incorrect. This ethnic group is, in fact, much less likely to have head lice than other races.

Head lice have claws that are adapted for grasping on to hairs, but the shape and width of African American hair renders this adaptation virtually useless. The lice literally cannot attach themselves.

Since hair texture varies from individual to individual, however, it is certainly possible for any person of any ethnicity to be subject to the presence of head lice, but this is much less likely with African Americans.

Head Lice and Disease

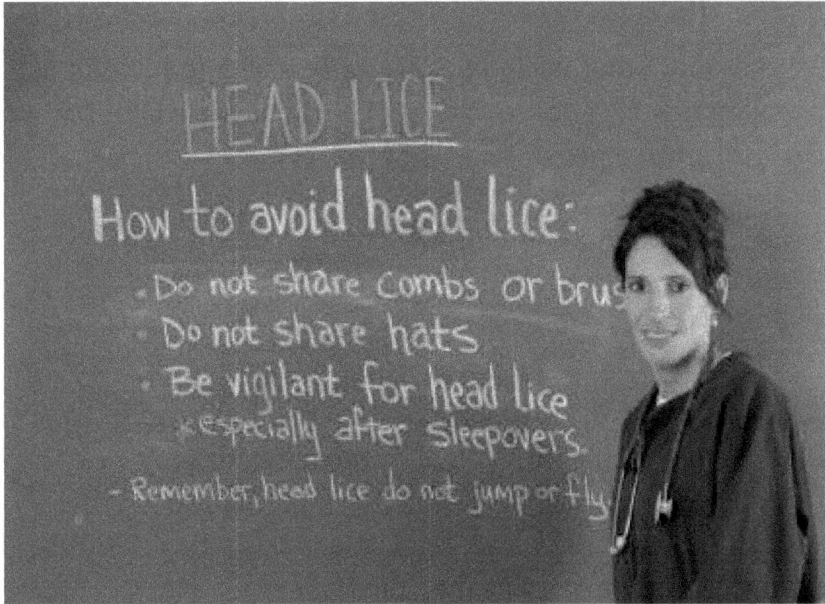

Although there is a strong cultural and hygenic reaction to the presence of head lice, the parasites can, but do not always spread disease.

Conventional medicine insists that only body lice are associated with the spread of pathogens. Head and pubic lice are considered to be uncomfortable annoyances, but they do not constitute a public health hazard.

Many parents object to their child's school conducting random inspections for the presence of head lice. This is not a reflection on the personal hygiene or even social standing of any given child.

Head lice are highly communicable, especially among children, but an infestation is also highly treatable.

Schools and other facilities are simply trying to prevent a problem before it occurs. Such inspections are a vital part of that preventive program.

Symptoms of Head Lice

The symptoms of head lice include:

- A crawling or tickling sensation on the scalp and in the hair created by the movement of the parasites.

- Itching as a result of an allergic reaction to the bites the lice inflict on the scalp as they feed.

- Open sores that form on the head due to scratching. Often these sores become infected from bacteria present on the skin.

A person with head lice will also be irritable and tired. The parasites are most active at night, which prevents the affected person from getting an adequate amount of rest.

Additionally, the constant itching causes a high level of discomfort and agitation.

Diagnosing Head Lice

The most reliable diagnosis of head lice is the visible identification of a living adult or nymph on the scalp or in the hair of the affected person. This can be difficult, however, for a number of reasons:

- The parasites are incredibly small.
- Lice and nymphs move quickly.
- They avoid the light.

Often a fine-tooth comb will be used to attempt to trap the lice for examination under a magnifying glass. It is also important to look for nits a quarter of an inch (0.64 cm) from the scalp, but these are hard to detect.

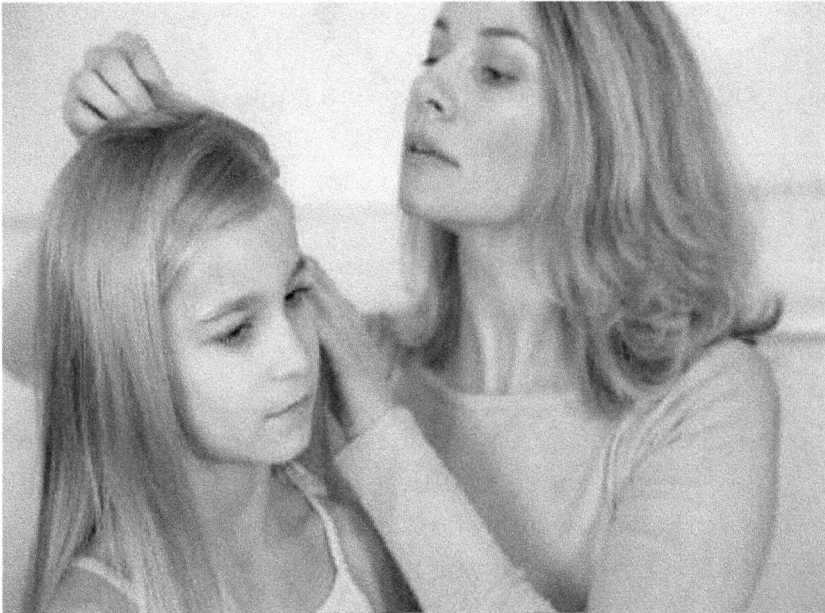

Part I – Understanding Head Lice

If you suspect you or your child have lice, it is strongly recommended that a qualified health care worker trained in the detection of the parasites make the final determination.

Treating Head Lice

When lice are found on one member of a household, all members should be immediately checked for the presence of the parasites.

All individuals with any sign of an active presence of lice should be treated. If two individuals share a bed, both should be treated, even if one does not immediately show signs of an active infestation.

Two types of lice-specific medications or pediculicides are widely used:

- Ovicidal prepartions that also kill the nits or eggs.

- Weak or non-ovicidal products that treat crawling adults.

If an ovicidal medicine is used, retreatment is only indicated if crawling adults are seen several days after the first dose is administered.

For appliations that are not ovicidal, repeat applications are strongly recommended. Multiple treatments may be necessary to get ahead of the cycle of hatching eggs and disrupt the self-perpetuating nature of the infestation.

Administer anti-lice preparations according to the instructions on the packaging. Read the directions carefully.

For individuals with long hair, it may be necessary to use twice the normal amount.

Make sure that the preparation remains in the hair for the recommended length of time. Additionally:

- Do NOT use a combination shampoo and conditioner medication on the hair prior to administering an anti-lice treatment.

- Do NOT wash the hair for 1-2 days after the lice medication has been rinsed.

If live, active lice are detected 8-12 hours after the treatment, consult with your health provider to determine if another pediculicide product may be needed.

Most of these products also include fine-toothed combs that are useful in dislodging nits and adults from the hair shaft. The comb should be used over a period of 2-3 weeks every 2-3 days to check for any signs of re-infestation.

(Note that some treatments do recommend a second application approximately 7-9 days after the initial use. Increasingly this is becoming a standard protocol. Again, always follow the instructions on the label precisely and do not use more than the indicated amount.)

Over-the-Counter Medications

The major anti-head lice treatments that can be purchased without a prescription include products that contain the following active ingredients.

Pyrethrins

The pyrethroid extracts from which pyrethrins are made are derived from chrysanthemums. Considered to be safe if used as directed, pyrethrin-based products will kill live adult lice, but not the unhatched eggs.

A second treatment is recommended on the 9th day to kill the next generation of hatched lice before they have an opportunity to lay more eggs.

If, however, you are allergic to either chrysanthemums or ragweed, these are not products you should use. Also, these products are not appropriate for children under 2 years of age.

One-Percent Permethrin Lotion

Permethrin lotion is a synthetic pyrethroid. Although products with permethrin will continue to kill newly hatched lice for several days after the initial application, a second treatment on the 9th day is still necessary.

Like natural pyrethroids, permethrin cannot be used on childen younger than 2 years of age.

Prescription Medications

The major treatments that are available and that require a prescription include the following preparations.

Five-Percent Benzyl Alcohol Lotion

Benzyl alcohol, an aromatic alcohol, will kill lice but not nits. Seven days after the initial application, a second treatment is required.

This product can be used with affected individuals age six months and older, but it may cause skin irritation, especially in older people.

Ivermectin Lotion (0.5%)

Ivermectin lotion can also be used in people age 6 months and older. It will not kill nits, but it does eliminate nymphs before they can mature.

The mixture is used as a single application on dry hair with no combing of nits required. (Many people do choose to comb the nits for aesthetic reasons, however. As long as the lotion itself is not removed before the indicated time, this is not a problem.)

It is important not to administer a second dosage of Ivermectin without the guidance of a medical professional as the lotion may not be well tolerated by all patients.

Malathion Lotion (0.5%)

The organophosphate malathion kills live lice and some lice eggs. A second application is still recommended 7-9 days after the first application.

This medication is recommended for affected individuals age 6 years and older, and may cause skin irritation. It is applied to wet hair.

Since the lotion is flammable, it is important not to apply it near a source of heat, including curlers and hair dryers, and not to smoke during the treatment.

Spinosad (0.9%)

Spinosad is a topical suspension made from soil bacteria. It kills live lice and nits. There is rarely a need for re-application. Spinosad may be used in individuals aged 4 years and older.

Retreatments are only indicated if live lice are detected one week after the first use.

Lindane Shampoo

Lindane is regarded as a "second line" treatment. It is an organochloride, but there are significant toxicity issues with its use.

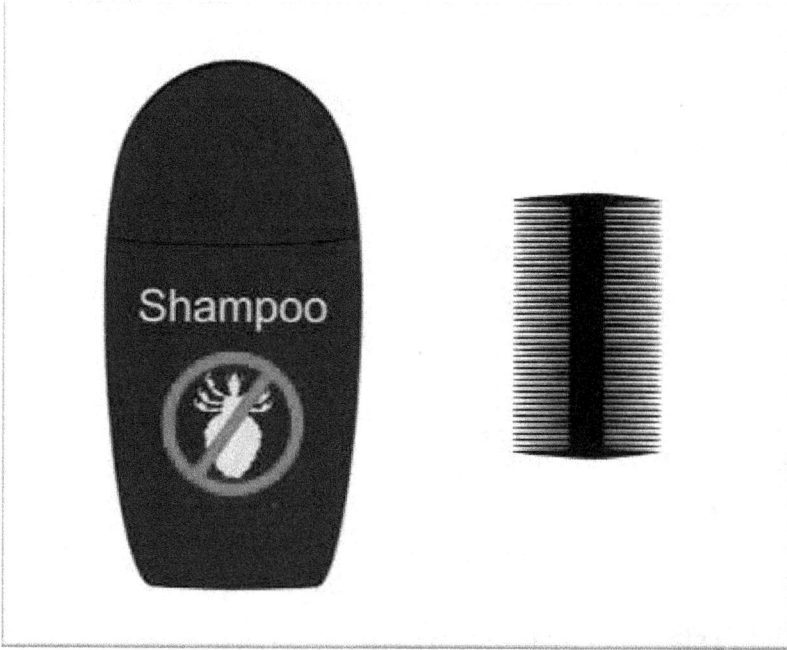

When used too aggressively or not as directed, Lindane can be toxic to the brain and nervous system. It should never be swallowed.

Currently Lindane is only used when other treatments have failed, or when the affected individual cannot tolerate other approaches.

Lindane should not be used with premature infants, infants, HIV patients, individuals with any kind of seizure disorder, women who are pregnant or breast-feeding, people with sores or irritated skin, the elderly, or anyone weighing less than 110 pounds (7.86 st).

Reapplication of Lindane should be avoided under all circumstances.

Supplementary Measures

Although supplementary measures are not technically required to stop an infestation of lice, these tactics carry a strong psychological benefit for the affected person and for others living in the home or using the same facility.

Any hats, scarves, articles of clothing, and bedding worn or used by the affected person in the 2 days before the discovery of the parasites should be machine washed in hot water and dried on a hot air cycle.

All life stages of head lice will die when exposed to temperatures of more than 128.3 F / 53.5 C for more than 5 minutes.

Any non-washable items should be sealed in a plastic bag for 2 weeks. Dry cleanable items should be cleaned and then sealed in plastic bags for at least 2 weeks.

Either boil (128.3 F / 53.5 C for 5 minutes) or throw out grooming aids like combs and brushes used by the affected person, and vacuum floors and furniture to remove loose hairs to which eggs might be attached.

Avoid the use of fumigant sprays. These products carry a high degree of toxicity, especially when inhaled or absorbed into the skin.

Part I – Understanding Head Lice

- Do not exceed the recommended amount of any head lice treatment unless directed to do so by a qualified medical health professional or a pharmacist.

- Be extremely careful to keep all medications away from the eyes. If contamination does occur, flush the eyes immediately with clean water.

- If a medication does not work after 2 to 3 treatments, discontinue and seek professional medical advice.

- Never mix anti-lice treatments, or use more than one treatment at a time.

- Do not use toxic fumigating sprays or fogs.

Preventing and Controlling Head Lice

The most frequently seen vector for the transmission of head lice is head-to-head contact. It is less common for an infestation to be linked to shared items of clothing, or from carpet and furniture.

These parasites can live no more than 2 days without a host. Nits will die within a week if they are not kept in an environment that mimics the temperature level and degree of humidity found on the human scalp.

Part I – Understanding Head Lice

The following steps will help to prevent head lice transmission and to control the spread of lice once the parasites are detected:

- During play, sporting events, and other activities at a facility where children are present in groups, avoid head-to-head contact.

- Do not allow for the sharing of articles of clothing. Particularly troublesome items include hats, caps, and scarves, coats, sports uniforms, and hair ribbons and barrettes.

- Do not allow personal care items like combs and brushes to be shared. If lice are detected these items must be disinfected in hot water of at least 128.3 F / 53.5 C for 5-10 minutes.

- Towels should not be shared, and should also be washed in 128.3 F / 53.5 C water if lice have been detected.

- There should be no contact with any form of bedding including pillows. This precaution also extends to couches, carpets, and stuffed animals.

- Items that cannot be washed or dry cleaned should be stored in a tightly sealed plastic bag for at least 2 weeks.

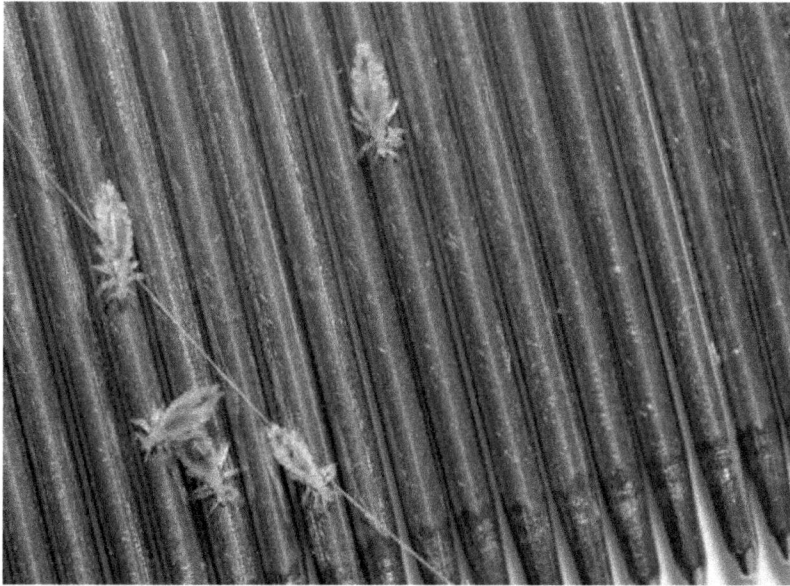

Reporting Head Lice

Although it is not required by law that a case of head lice be reported to the health authorities, it is important that this fact not be kept hidden out of shame or embarrassment.

Lice infestations are easily passed from person to person. Childcare workers, school nurses, other parents, facility directors, and other responsible individuals need to know that lice are present.

To completely eradicate the parasites, steps must be taken to rid the environment of surviving eggs. If this is not done, the infestation will continue to manifest regardless of the treatment or deterrents applied.

Part I – Understanding Head Lice

Part II – Understanding Body Lice

Adult body lice are 2.3 to 3.6 mm in length. These parasitic insects live in and lay eggs on clothing, moving to the skin of the infected person only when they are feeding on blood. Body lice are also typically found in bedding and towels.

Unlike head lice, body lice do spread diseases including:

- typhus
- relapsing fever
- trench fever

The most common vector for transmission of an infestation of lice is person-to-person contact, most often in crowded conditions where the hygiene is poor. Examples might include the homeless or refugees. Animals do not spread any form of human lice.

The parasites are found around the world among all races. Like head lice, they pass through three life stages: nit or egg, nymph and adult.

Symptoms of Body Lice

The most common symptom indicating the presence of body lice is severe itching accompanies by a rash caused by allergic skin reactions to the bites.

When the infested person begins to scratch, open sores typically develop and become infected due to the presence of bacteria on the skin.

In long-standing cases of body lice, the skin will darken and become thicker. This effect is most pronounced on the mid-section and is commonly referred to as "vagabond's disease."

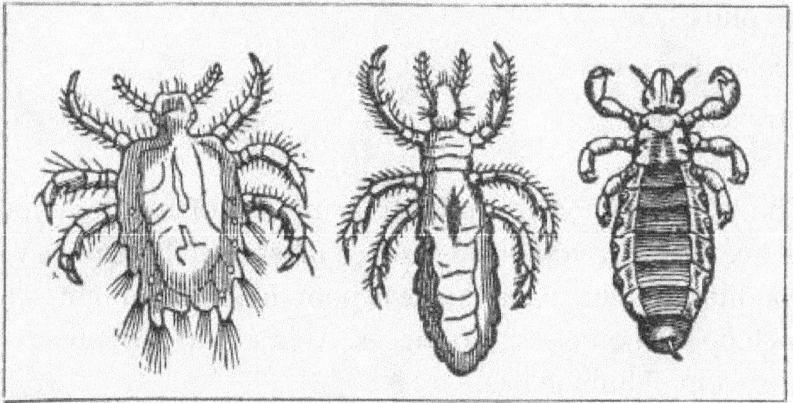

Diagnosis of Body Lice

Cases of body lice are diagnosed by visual identification of adults crawling and feeding on the skin, and by the presence of adults and eggs in the seams of clothing and bedding.

It may be necessary to use a means of magnification to properly determine if the parasites are present.

Treating Body Lice

The only treatment that is needed to cure body lice infestation is access to clean clothes on a weekly basis and better personal hygiene.

When a person is found to be infested with body lice, their clothing, bedding, and towels should be washed in water that is at least 128.3 F / 53.5 C and dried on the hottest machine cycle available.

Typically the use of a pediculicide treatment agent is not necessary.

Preventing and Controlling Body Lice

Body lice spread via person-to-person contact among populations living in close proximity with little to no access to clean clothing and bathing facilities. All of the following steps can be used to prevent and/or control an infestation of body lice:

- Make sure the population in question has an opportunity to bathe regularly and has access to clean, parasite-free clothing at least once a week.

- Infested clothing and bedding should be washed and dried at temperatures of 128.3 F / 53.5 C or above.

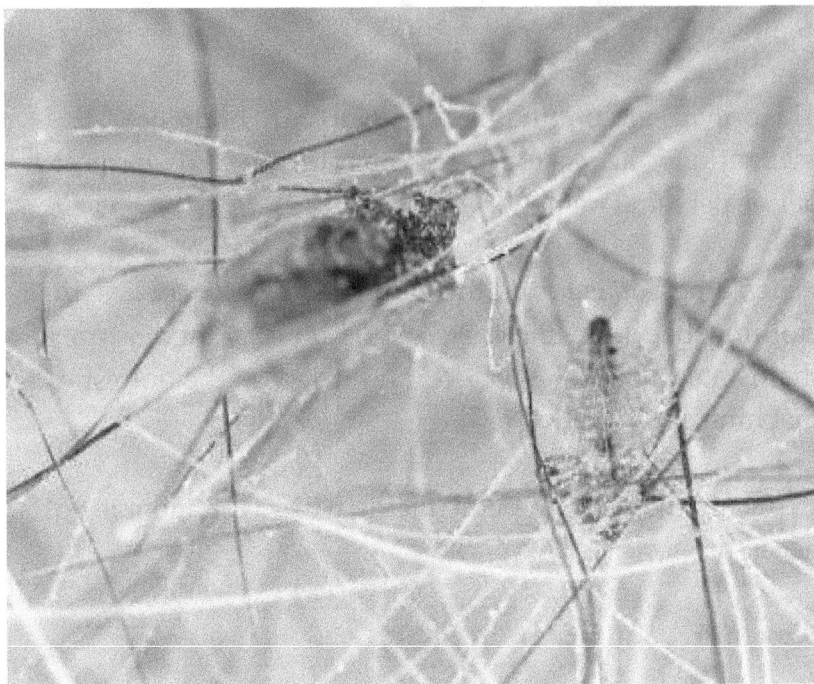

- Any items that cannot be washed or dry cleaned should be sealed in a plastic bag and stored for a minimum of two weeks.

- Individuals living in crowded conditions with limited hygiene options should not share clothing, bedding, or towels.

Note that it is sometimes necessary to use dusting chemicals or fumigating agents to control body lice if there is a danger of an epidemic disease like typhus spreading.

Part III – Understanding Pubic Lice

Adult pubic lice are 1.1-1.8 mm in length and infest the hair in the pubic area, occasionally spreading to coarse hair on other parts of the body, for instance beards or eyebrows.

An infestation is properly called pthiriasis, but is commonly referred to as having "crabs." The name derives from the over-sized nature of the first two legs on the parasite, which resemble a crab's pinchers.

Pubic lice are typically spread via sexual contact. Pets do not play a role in the transmission of the lice.

Pubic lice are found around the world and there is no association with specific races, ethnic, or socio-economic groups. Because the parasites are spread by sexual contact, infestations are seen most commonly in children.

If pubic lice are found in children, the fact is almost a certain indicator of sexual abuse.

The lice do not themselves transmit diseases, but due to the severe itching they cause, secondary bacterial infections are possible where the skin breaks down because of scratching.

Diagnosing Pubic Lice

Pubic lice are diagnosed by a visual inspection that reveals the presence of adults or nits in the pubic hair. The parasites may be visible to the naked eye, but magnification may be necessary to confirm the diagnosis.

Typically when an individual is found to be infested with pubic lice, they are immediately evaluated for other sexually transmitted diseases.

Treating Pubic Lice

Over-the-counter medications containing one of the following agents are often used to treat an infestation of pubic lice:

- 1% permethrin
- pyrethrins
- piperonyl butoxide

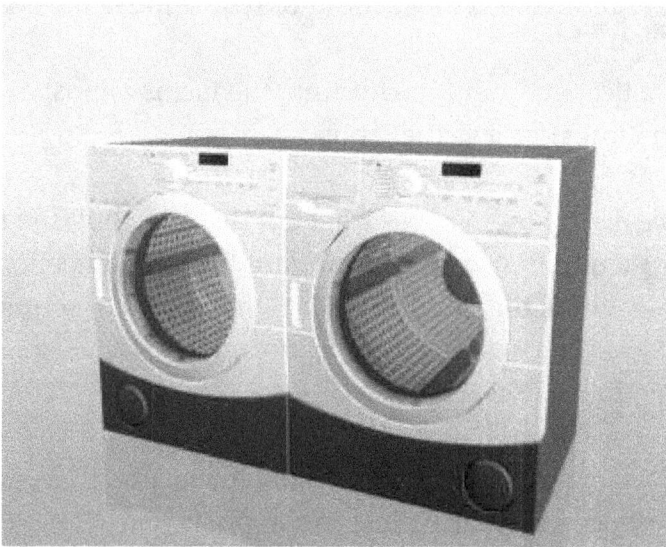

Part III – Understanding Pubic Lice

When used exactly as directed, these products are considered to be safe and effective. The infested area should be washed thoroughly and dried before the pubic hair is saturated with the treatment agent.

Always leave the product in place for the recommended time and remove the treatment agent in the manner directed. As the nits or eggs will remain attached to the hair shafts, they must be removed, generally with a fine-toothed comb.

Understand that it may be necessary to perform a second treatment in 9-10 days if live lice are still present.

Clean underwear and clothing should be worn post-treatment, with the previous clothing laundered in water at a minimum temperature of 128.3 F / 53.5 C and dried at the hottest cycle available.

Any items that cannot be washed or dry cleaned should be sealed in plastic bags for two weeks.

If pubic lice are present in the eyebrows or eyelashes, it may be possible to control the infestation with a fine-toothed comb only.

An opthalmic-grade petroleum ointment may be required, however, and can only be obtained via a prescription. Over-the-counter petroleum jelly should not be used.

Part III – Understanding Pubic Lice

Prescription treatments for pubic lice could include:

- Lindane shampoo
- Malathion lotion
- Ivermectin

Lindane is not considered to be a first-line treatment due to its potential toxicity for the brain and nervous system. It is most often prescribed only in patients where other treatments have not proved to be effective. Lindane should not be used with:

- premature infants
- infants
- children
- the elderly
- individuals afflicted with a seizure-inducing disorder
- pregnant or breast-feeding women
- anyone with severely irritate skin
- individuals who weigh 110 pounds (7.86 st) or less

Malathion and Ivermectin can both kill lice and some eggs, but it is not routinely used for pubic lice.

Inform Sexual Partners

All sexual partners of the infested individual during the previous 30 days should be informed of the diagnosis of pubic lice as they, too, will require treatment. These individuals should also be evaluated for the presence of other sexually transmitted diseases.

Preventing and Controlling Pubic Lice

Pubic lice are rarely spread via clothing, bedding, or a toilet seat. The common vector of transmission is sexual contact. Once the presence of pubic lice has been detected, all the individual's sexual partners must be informed.

Abstinence from sexual activity until the infestation has been cured is crucial to prevent the spread of the parasites. All clothing and bedding should be washed at 128.3 F / 53.5 C or above. Items that cannot be laundered should be sealed in plastic bags for two weeks.

Do not use fogs or fumigation products as these agents are toxic if absorbed through the skin or inhaled.

Quick Facts – Lice

- Lice do not jump like fleas, nor can they fly. They are biting insects, not burrowing.

- One thing that makes lice difficult to detect is their natural tendency to hide from the light. Lice are so tiny, they are often mistaken for dandruff — until you see one moving!

- Because lice are most active at night, people suffering from an infestation tend to be cranky from lack of sleep as well as the intense itching the parasites cause.

- Lice are best adapted to grasping fine, straight hair. This means that African Americans are actually less likely to have head lice.

- When absent a human host, lice cannot survive for more than 24-48 hours.

- On the human head, an adult louse can live for 30 days.

- Female lice are capable of laying 6 eggs per day.

- Although there is some debate about the matter, head lice are not believed to transmit disease. Body lice, however, can spread typhus and relapsing fever.

- Swimming will not kill lice as the insects can survive for 8 hours under water.

Quick Facts – Lice

- Lice are so good at hanging on to hairs with their claws that a vigorous washing alone is not enough to get rid of the parasites.

- A head lice infestation is not an indication of poor personal hygiene, in fact, lice prefer clean hair shafts, which are easier to grip.

- Body lice do tend to proliferate in crowded conditions where hygiene is poor.

- Pubic lice are called crabs because their front legs have enlarged pinchers.

- Since pubic lice are primarily spread by sexual contact, their presence on a child is an indicator of sexual abuse.

- Lice are not a new problem for humans. The first confirmed connection between lice and humans was 10,000 years ago!

- Lice are species specific. Dogs and cats can get lice, but those lice have no interest in attaching themselves to humans.

Part IV – Understanding Scabies

A microscopic, burrowing, parasitic mite, *Sarcoptes scabiei var. hominis*, causes human scabies. The creatures are often referred to as the "human itch mite."

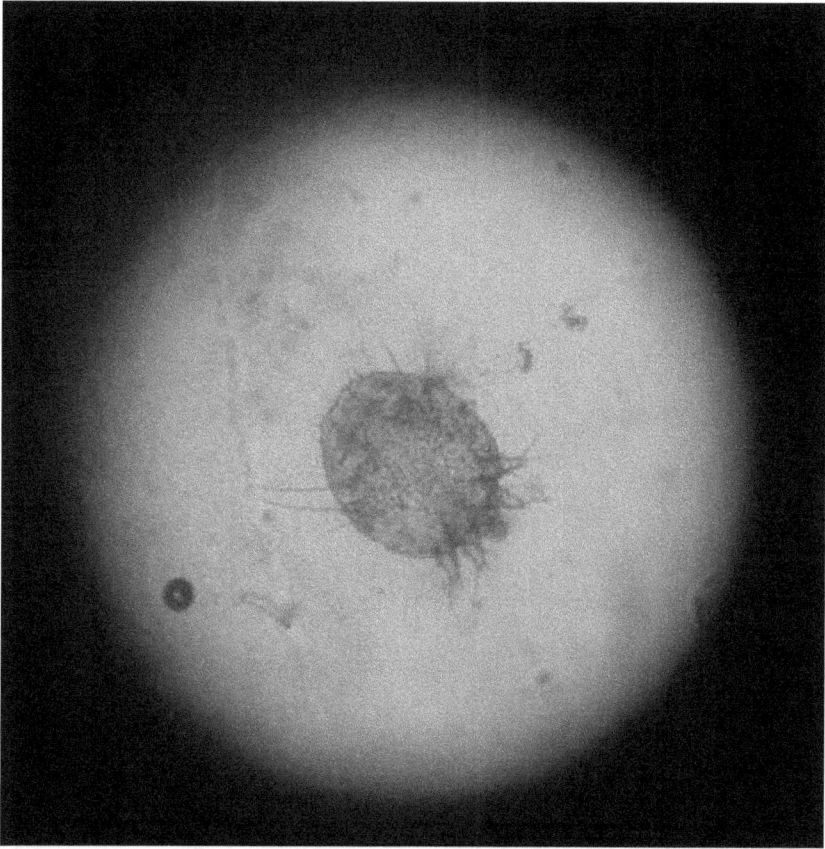

Other species of scabies mites can cause infestations in mammals including dogs and cats. Humans who come into contact with affected animals may develop a dermatitis like rash that will be self-limiting, but the mites will not thrive and breed on a human host.

The human scabies mites infest and lay their eggs in the upper skin layer causing a pimpled skin rash and intense itching. The burrows have a distinctive, serpentine appearance on the skin and may be flesh toned or gray.

Scabies Mite Lifecycle

The human scabies mite pass through a four-stage lifecycle:

- egg
- larva
- nymph
- adult

As female mites burrow, they can lay 2-3 oval eggs per day that are 0.10-0.15 mm in length. The eggs hatch in 3-4 days, with the larvae migrating to the surface of the skin where they create short burrows called molting pouches.

After 3-4 days the larvae molt and become nymphs, which also live in molting pouches or attach themselves to hair follicles. They mature into round adult mites that have the appearance of sacs and lack eyes.

Females are 0.30-0.45 mm long and 0.25-0.35 mm wide. Males are approximately half that size. Males and females mate one time, after which the female is fertile for the remainder of her life.

Once impregnated, females find a site to dig a permanent burrow to lay her eggs over the course of the next 1-2 months. Approximately 10% of the eggs will produce new adult mites.

Scabies Transmission

The parasites spread via prolonged direct skin-to-skin contact and can be passed along by persons who have no obvious symptoms. Animals play no role in spreading scabies among humans.

Scabies infestations are seen in all parts of the world, and are not specific to any ethnic group or socio-economic class. The mites do spread rapidly, however, in overcrowded conditions like:

- prisons
- nursing homes
- extended care facilities

It is also quite common for scabies to be spread by sexual contact, or to be passed around among members of the same household.

In institutional settings, especially in cases of virulent crusted scabies, prevention hinges on vigilant monitoring and detection once the outbreak has been identified.

If crusted scabies is present, this will include a program of thorough cleaning and disinfecting in addition to treating the affected individuals.

Since direct skin-to-skin contact is the means of transmission, affected individuals may need to be temporarily isolated and support staff will require protective garments.

Crusted (Norwegian) Scabies

Crusted or Norwegian Scabies is a more serious form of the disease with large numbers of adult mites and eggs present — as many as 2 million per patient. Individuals with this condition are considered highly contagious and require fast and aggressive medical treatment.

At-risk populations include:

- elderly individuals
- the disabled or debilitated
- immunocompromised persons

Anyone with loss of sensation or movement can be subject to this more virulent form of infestation.

Skin-to-skin contact is not the only transmission vector in cases of crusted scabies, which can also be spread by mites that have been shed into clothing or bedding or fallen onto furniture.

Rooms used by infested individuals must be thoroughly cleaned and vacuumed, but pesticide spray, fogs, and fumigants are discouraged due to their high level of toxicity.

Symptoms of Scabies Infestation

After a person becomes infested with scabies, symptoms do not appear for 2-6 weeks. During that time, the individual can spread the mites to other humans. Common symptoms include:

- severe itching, particularly at night when the mites are most active

- a pimple-like, itchy rash

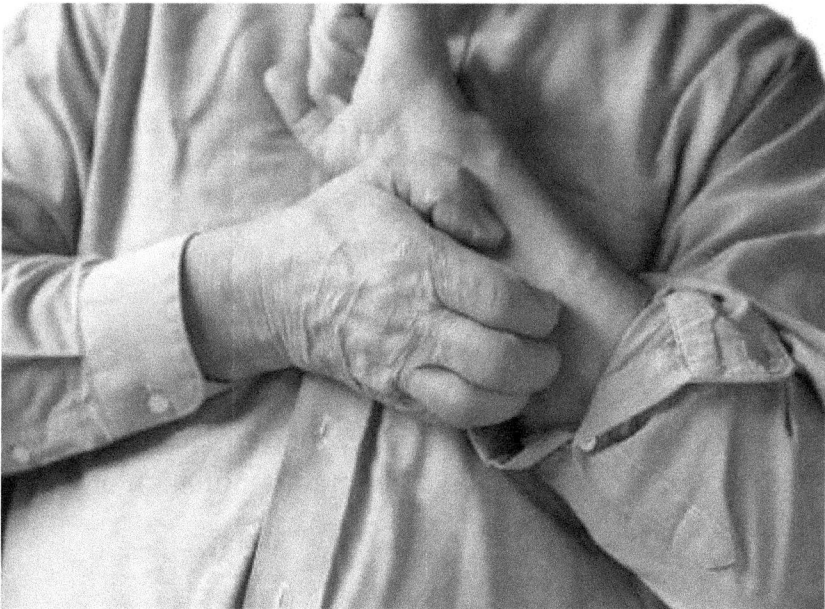

Part IV – Understanding Scabies

The most common sites for the scabies rash to be present include:

- between the fingers
- on the wrist
- at the elbow
- in the armpit
- around the nipples
- at the waist
- on the buttocks
- over and between the shoulder blades

In infants, scabies is often seen on the head, neck, and face, as well as the palms of the hands and the soles of the feet.

Potential Complications

Due to the severe itching caused by an infestation of scabies mites, the affected person often scratches until skin sores develop. It is not unusual for the sores to become infected with bacteria including:

- Staphylococcus aureus
- Beta-hemolytic streptococci

It is possible for a bacterial skin infection to cause post-streptococcal glomerulonephritis, an inflammation of the kidneys.

Part IV – Understanding Scabies

Diagnosis of Scabies

The distinctive appearance of the scabies burrows makes visual diagnoses highly reliable, but typically the mite will be removed from the end of the burrow with a tip of a needle or a skin scraping will be taken to confirm the diagnosis.

A diagnosis can still be difficult, however, especially when the mites, their eggs, or their droppings are not detectable under the microscope.

Infested individuals may have no more than 10-15 mites present on their bodies.

Treating and Preventing Scabies

The treatment products use with scabies are called "scabicides." Most kill the adult mites, and some address the eggs as well.

There are no over-the-counter preparations to cure scabies. All treatments must be prescribed by a doctor. These include:

- 5% permethrin cream, which can be used from the age of 2 months forward

- 10% Crotamiton lotion or cream, which is an adult medication

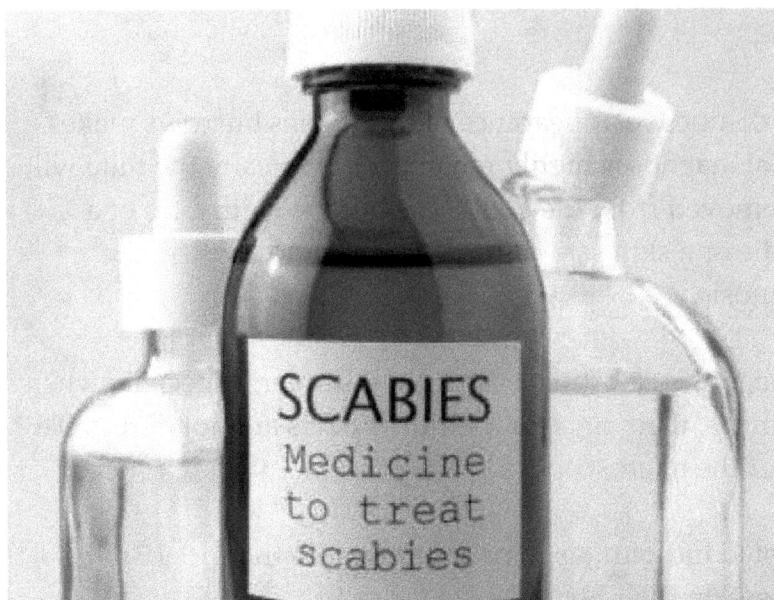

In highly resistant cases, Lindane lotion may be used. The medication is, however, potentially toxic to the brain and nervous system.

The use of Lindane is dangerous to given populations including infants, the elderly, pregnant and nursing women, and individuals weighing less than 110 pounds (7.86 st), it is considered a strategy of last resort.

Ivermectin, which is typically a treatment for worm infestations, may be a safe and effective treatment for scabies when taken orally, but this is not yet regarded as a standard approach.

The medications most typically dispensed are permethrin or Crotamiton lotions or creams. They must be applied to the entire body. In babies, this includes the entire head and all regions of the neck and face.

Treatments should be applied to a clean body only, and left on for the length of time indicated on the directions. Clean clothing must always be worn post-treatment.

Scabies mites do not survive longer than 2-3 days off human skin. All clothing, bedding, and towels used by the affected person or by their sexual partners or household members must be thoroughly washed in hot water and dried on the highest available setting.

Anything that cannot be washed or dry cleaned should be sealed in a plastic bag for at least 72 hours. Skin-to-skin contact must be avoided as soon as the infestation is identified and until it has been conclusively resolved.

The severe itching that is the hallmark of a scabies infestation are caused by a hyper-allergic skin reaction. The itching may not stop immediately after a treatment, and can go on for another 2-4 weeks.

It is important, however, to watch for the development of any new burrows or rashes, which would mean a second course of treatment is needed.

Part IV – Understanding Scabies

Quick Facts - Scabies

- Scabies is a condition caused by a burrowing skin parasite called the human itch mite.

- Symptoms of scabies may take 4-6 weeks to develop. During that time, the affected person can transmit the mites to others.

- The mites that cause scabies can live up to 2 days absent a human host.

- Crusted or Norwegian scabies is a virulent type of infestation with thousands of mites present. It requires stringent containment protocols and vigorous medical intervention.

- Scabies is not a reflection on the quality of personal hygiene. It's spread by direct contact. Anyone can pick up the human itch mite.

- Scabies is not a sexually transmitted disease, although sexual contact is often the vector for an infestation.

- There are no over-the-counter treatments for scabies. Prescription medications from a doctor are necessary to combat the infestation.

- Contrary to urban myth, scabies can be cured. It is not a chronic or life-long condition.

Quick Facts - Scabies

- Severe, relentless itching is the major symptom of scabies, which often leads to the development of open sores from scratching. These can easily become infected.

Natural Remedies for Lice and Scabies

Although over-the-counter and prescription anti-lice treatments are regarded as safe if used as directed, many people are reluctant to use chemical products, especially with children.

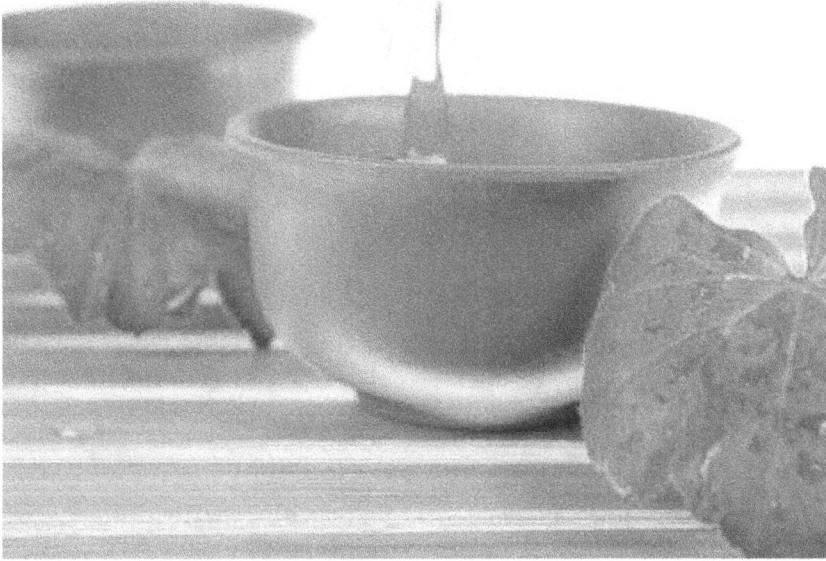

Natural Remedies for Lice

The following alternative treatments are all geared at treating head lice infestations.

A Fine-Toothed Nit Comb

Even chemical-based lice remedies typically include a fine-toothed comb (often called a "nit comb") in their packaging.

Using one of these combs is the most effective way to elminiate lice eggs at the base of the hair shaft and to remove live, crawling lice in dry hair.

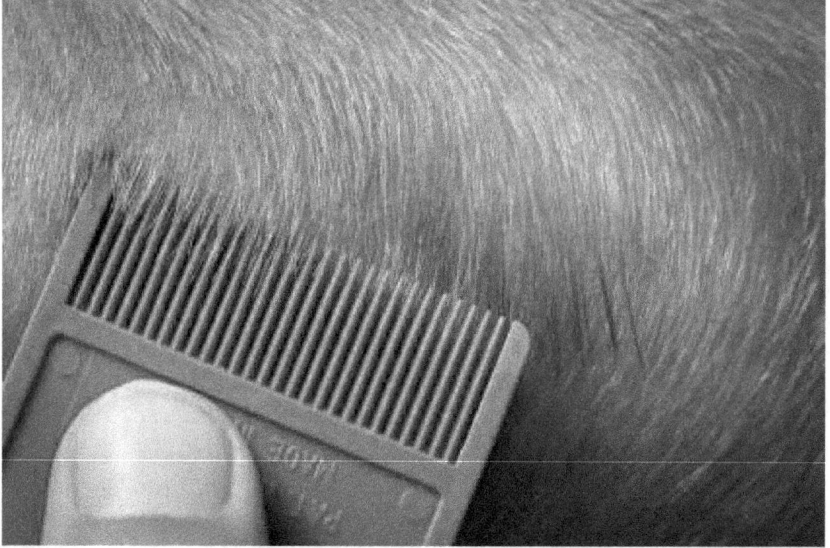

The method is even more effective if a light coating of tea tree oil is applied to the comb periodically during the treatment.

Clean out the comb by soaking it in vinegar for half an hour or by boiling it for 5-10 minutes. Repeat three times a day for the first week and nightly for the second week.

Tea Tree Oil

Tea tree oil is an effective natural insecticide and can be easily mixed with natural shampoos at a ratio of 3-5 drops per one ounce (U.S. or UK).

Natural Remedies for Lice and Scabies

As an alternative, mix a teaspoon (U.S. or UK) of tea tree oil with about 3 tablespoons (U.S. or UK) of a carrier oil in a bowl and apply to the hair for 30-45 minutes before shampooing with any normal product.

(Although it's not necessary for the treatment to be effective, warming the oil slightly makes the process much more enjoyable.)

Appropriate carrier oils include:

- olive
- jojoba
- sesame
- coconut

You can also use 10-20 drops of tea tree oil per load of wash to treat items suspected of carrying lice.

Neem Oil

Neem oil is also a natural insecticide that is a favorite with gardeners. Shampoos that include neem oil are available in health food stores, or you can simply add a few teaspoons (U.S. or UK) to your regular shampoo.

There is no set formula, just work for a consistency that is even and not overly oily.

Natural Remedies for Lice and Scabies

Additional Oil Treatments

There are numerous oils that can be used in combination or individually to treat infestations of head lice. Any time you are applying an oil treatment, it's a good idea to first rinse the hair with apple cider vinegar and allow it to dry.

Nits attach themselves with a substance that is very like glue. The acidic nature of the vinegar weakens this bond and helps the heavier oils to remove the lice eggs.

For an overnight oil treatment use the following recipe (measurements can be either US or UK):

- 1/4 cup sesame seed oil
- 1/8 cup neem oil
- 1 teaspoon tea tree oil
- 1/2 teaspoon eucalyptus oil
- 1/2 teaspoon rosemary oil
- 10 drops lavendar oil

Apply this mixture to the hair and scalp. Cover the head with a shower cap and leave in place 6-8 hours, then use a fine-toothed comb to remove dead lice and nits.

A straight application of coconut oil after an apple cider vinegar rinse is especially effective as well, particularly if you add a few drops of ylang-ylang and anise oils.

Natural Remedies for Lice and Scabies

The Goals of Alternative Treatments

The point of most of these applications is to suffocate the living lice and to create a heavy carrier base for nits to be combed out of the hair.

Many of these essential oils have antibacterial, anti-inflammatory, and antibiotic properties, however. They work to soothe the irritation to the scalp created by the lice bites, and to lessen the chance of secondary infections from scratching.

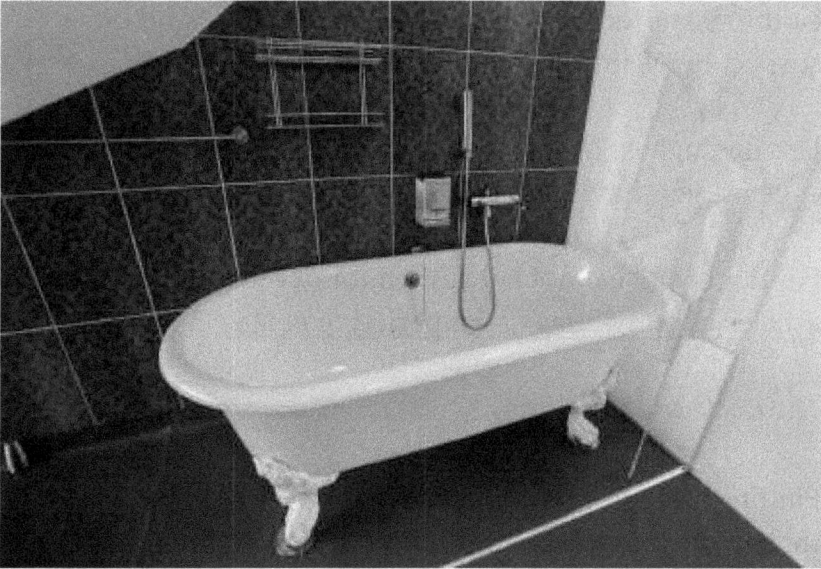

Some applications are also thought to discourage additional lice activity because the insects are repelled by the strong smell of the preparation.

Natural Remedies for Lice and Scabies

An example of a very strong smelling application is garlic paste created by grinding 8-10 cloves of garlic mixed with 2-3 teaspoons (US or UK) of lime juice and 10-15 drops of tea tree oil.

The paste should be left in for half an hour and then rinsed thoroughly. Be forewarned, however, that even with a thorough rinsing, the garlic odor will linger in the hair.

Washing Exposed Items

All of these treatments should be paired with washing all clothing, stuffed animals, linens, hats, towels, and other suspect items in water that is at least 128.3 F / 53.5 C.

Use the highest dryer setting possible to be sure any lice or eggs present have been killed.

For items that cannot be washed (or dry cleaned), seal the articles in plastic bags for a period of at least 2 weeks.

Natural Remedies for Scabies

Finding a natural remedy for scabies is somewhat harder than treating lice. The most popular remedy that can be used for both is tea tree oil. It appears to be the most effective at penetrating the skin and suffocating the parasites.

This is similar to the home remedy of using nail polish to eradicate chiggers. Don't try this with scabies, however, as the mites simply relocate as the polish is drying.

Cayenne Bath

A more aggressive treatment for scabies is to spend an extended amount of time in a warm bath mixed with cayenne. Be very cautious to protect your eyes from being splashed with the pepper. The cayenne will literally burn the mites without causing any health problems.

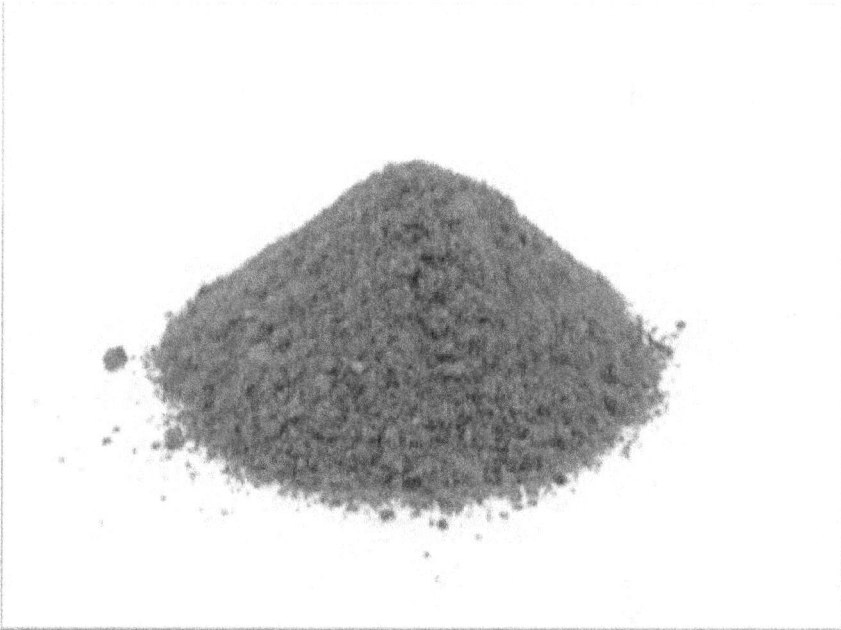

There is no set amount of cayenne to use, simply mix the pepper powder into the water as you would a bath salt

Natural Remedies for Lice and Scabies

Neem Oil and Soap

Neem oil will also prevent the mites from reproducing, and after two days, people suffering with scabies no longer seem to be getting bitten.

There will still be adult mites alive on the body, however, so if you use neem, you will want to apply it over the whole body and if possible shower daily with neem soap for two weeks.

Zinc

Zinc cream is very useful to help to prevent or to treat secondary skin infections that develop as a consequence of scratching. This will also guard against fungal infections that can opportunistically break out.

You can make your own cream or paste by crushing zinc tablets and mixing in some turmeric, which will help to stop itching. The turmeric also has anti-parasitic qualities.

Afterword

Far from being tied to any one race or socio-economic group, lice and scabies are simply highly efficient parasites that, when given a vector to exploit, will infest human beings to feed on our blood.

The parasites tend to thrive in crowded conditions. Some are benign like daycare facilities, elementary schools, and nursing homes, while others are tied to disaster and trauma like refugee camps and homeless populations.

Most infestations are spread by skin-to-skin contact, while body lice and scabies can be transmitted via articles of clothing and bedding. In the case of body lice, poor hygiene is a factor, but with head lice, the infestation is not a reflection of personal or environmental cleanliness.

Because people find the topic so distasteful, there is a great body of urban legend and myth built up around the action of these nuisance parasites. In truth, only body lice are clearly associated with the spread of disease.

All forms of lice and scabies can be treated. There are effective over-the-counter anti-lice products available, but scabies treatments must be prescribed by a doctor. When used as directed, these preparations will eradicate the parasites and are safe for use even with children.

The spread of the parasites can be controlled with vigorous washing and dry cleaning at high temperatures or tightly

Afterword

sealing items in plastic bags for a recommended period of time.

The purpose of this text has been to explain each of the parasites, their causes, the means of their transmission, the symptoms they cause, the recommended methods for treatments, and the protocols for their eradication.

With the exception of body lice, the greatest risk is of secondary skin infections caused by vigorous scratching in the presence of intense itching. When viewed absent of panic or recoil, lice and scabies are easily detected, cured, and eradicated.

Relevant Websites

The National Pediculosis Association, Inc.
www.headlice.org

Centers for Disease Control
www.cdc.gov/parasites/lice/

The Mayo Clinic Lice Information
www.mayoclinic.com/health/lice/DS00368

Information on Head Lice
www.headlice.org/

American Academy of Dermatology
www.aad.org

Head Lice
www.aad.org/skin-conditions/dermatology-a-to-z/lice

Scabies
www.aad.org/search/?k=scabies

Healthy Children
www.healthychildren.org

Relevant Websites

Frequently Asked Questions – Head Lice

Although it is recommended that you read the entire text regarding head lice, the following are some of the most frequently asked questions about the diagnosis, treatment, and eradication of these parasites.

What are head lice?

Head lice are parasites that infest the human hair, eyebrows and eyelashes where they feed on blood next to the scalp or skin. They do not spread disease, but they do cause extreme itching and often open sores develop as a result of incessant scratching.

Who gets head lice the most?

Head lice can be found anywhere in the world, but they are most common in groups of people that live or work in close quarters. In the United States, for instance, children are at the greatest risk in pre-schools and elementary schools.

It's a myth that lice are more prevalent in any one ethnic group. The parasites are found less frequently in African-Americans, for instance, because the lice cannot efficiently grasp the thicker hair shafts typical in this racial group.

Since lice cannot hop or fly transmission must occur by direct contact. Occasionally articles of clothing, personal grooming items, or sports gear are the means of transportation if human hairs have become detached and lodged in the items.

Hygiene and cleanliness either in the home or at the facility have no effect on the presence of lice.

What do head lice look like?

Lice have a three stage life cycle that begins with small, oval-shaped nits or eggs that are attached at the base of the hair shaft. The nits are no bigger than a knot in a piece of thread. They may be yellow or white, and are easily mistaken for dandruff. The eggs hatch in 8-9 days.

An immature louse is called a nymph. At this stage, the parasite needs blood to live. In 9-12 days, nymphs become adults that will live for 30 days. If they fall off the human host, they die in 2 days. Adults are tan to grayish-white, about the size of a sesame seed, and have six legs.

Where on the head are the lice most commonly found?

It's common to find lice concentrated behind the ears, and along the neckline at the back of the head.

What are the symptoms of an infestation of head lice?

The lice create a tickling sensation in the hair as they crawl. Their bites cause an allergic reaction on the scalp that leads to itching and in turn, scratching, especially at night when they are most active.

Lack of sleep will cause irritability in the person suffering from the infestation. The more the affected person scratches, the greater the chance that sores will develop on the scalp.

How is an infestation of head lice diagnosed?

The most definitive diagnosis is visual, finding a living nymph or adult on the scalp or in the hair. The parasites are very small and fast, however, and they avoid the light. Typically a fine-tooth comb and a magnifying glass are used as diagnostic aids.

Although it is possible to see the nits attached at the base of the hair shaft, it's easy to mistake them for dandruff, scabs, or even drops of hairspray. It's best to have a health care professional trained in the identification of lice examine the scalp to make an accurate diagnosis.

Is it necessary to report lice to some official entity?

Health departments and other agencies typically do not require that infestations of lice be reported, however, you should inform the school or facility administration if lice are detected so that control measures can be taken.

Do head lice spread disease?

No, head lice do not spread disease. They are an annoyance, and it is possible for a secondary infection to develop on the scalp from the scratching, but in and of themselves, head lice are not a health hazard.

Can sharing sports helmets and items like headphones spread lice?

It is uncommon for head lice to be spread by objects and personal belongings. The lice are physically adapted to hold on to human hair, therefore they cannot easily attach themselves to smooth surfaces.

Can lice spread through hair pieces and wigs?

Lice die quickly without a human host. Adults cannot live more than 2 days without feeding, and nymphs can survive only a few hours. Nits (eggs) will die within a week since they cannot hatch at temperatures lower than that of the human scalp. Consequently, it is extremely unlikely that a wig or hairpiece that has not been worn for at least 48 hours could transmit an infestation of lice.

Can lice be spread in swimming pools?

Although head lice can live underwater for several hours, transmission in a swimming pool is unlikely. Even when submerged, the lice don't turn lose of the hair shaft.

It is possible, though unlikely, for lice to be spread via towels and personal grooming items like combs and brushes, so it's best not to share those items.

It is a myth that the chlorine in swimming pool water will kill lice, however, swimming or even washing the hair 1-2 days after an anti-lice treatment has been used may render the application ineffective.

Are there specific lice treatment recommendations for different age groups?

It's always best to consult with your doctor before treating young children with any over-the-counter product. There may be specific cautions necessary in regard not just to the child's age and weight, but also to their personal medical history.

Do anti-lice treatments have any side effects?

If used as directed, over-the-counter and prescription treatments for head lice infestations are safe and effective. Because the scalp will likely be inflamed both from the bites and the scratching, feeling a mild burning sensation is typical.

Do all the nits have to be removed for the treatment to be effective?

Anti-lice medications are typically designed to be administered in two treatments. The second is to address any nymphs that have hatched after the first application. Nit removal is not necessary for a successful eradication of the parasites, but may be desirable for aesthetic reasons.

Why should some items be bagged for 2 weeks to kill lice?

Lice eggs or nits have to incubate at the temperature and humidity levels found on human scalp. It is highly unlikely that eggs will hatch absent a host, and without a supply of blood, nymphs will die within a few hours.

If, however, some personal items cannot be laundered or dry cleaned and there is a concern that eggs might be present, securely sealing them in plastic bags for two weeks will ensure that no lice, regardless of life stage, survive.

Should I treat my pets for head lice?

No, head lice don't live on pets, and animals don't play a role in spreading infestations of head lice.

Will household sprays kill grown lice?

It is not recommended that any sprays or fumigating products be used to combat an infestation of head lice. These items are highly toxic and they are not necessary. They should not be used on human beings, and it is not necessary to fumigate the premises.

Routine cleaning and laundering is more than sufficient to address potential spread of lice. The parasites cannot survive without a human host for more than 48 hours. Bag any items about which you have a concern and leave them sealed in plastic for two weeks.

Do I need to hire a pest control company to spray the house?

A pest control company is not necessary. No sprays or fumigating products are indicated to control an infestation of head lice, either over-the-counter or professionally applied.

Will regular laundering kill living lice on clothing and bedding?

Both washing and drying items at temperatures of more than 128.3 F / 53.5 C will kill head lice and their eggs. Dry cleaning has the same effect. Freezing temperatures are not as effective and should not be used as a treatment or eradication approach.

Frequently Asked Questions - Body Lice

Although it is recommended that you read the entire text regarding body lice, the following are some of the most frequently asked questions about the diagnosis, treatment, and eradication of these parasites.

What are body lice?

Body lice are parasites that live on clothing and bedding, typically laying their eggs in the seams. They feed on the blood of the affected person, and spread rapidly in crowded conditions where poor hygiene is a problem. For this reason, body lice are often seen among homeless populations, refugees, and victims of war.

What do body lice look like?

Like all forms of lice, body lice have three life stages: nit (egg), nymph, and adult. The eggs take 1-2 weeks to hatch. They are oval and yellowish white in color. The immature nymphs mature in 9-12 days, with the adults reaching the size of a sesame seed. They are gray to tan and have six legs.

Where can body lice typically be found?

Body lice will be found in both the clothing and bedding of people afflicted with an infestation. They lay their eggs in the seams of the fabric, and will sometimes attach themselves to body hair. Lice found on the head and scalp, however, are specific head lice.

What are the symptoms of an infestation of body lice?

People affected by an infestation of body lice will experience intense itching, and may have open and infected sores from scratching.

If the infestation is of long duration, the skin in areas that have been repeatedly bitten will become thick and discolored. This happens particularly in the midsection on the upper thighs, groin, and waist, a condition referred to as "vagabond's disease."

Do body lice transmit disease?

Body lice can be responsible for transmitting typhus, trench fever, and louse-borne relapsing fever. Outbreaks of typhus are no longer widely seen, but can occur during wartime, civil unrest, disasters, and in overcrowded, unsanitary prisons. Typhus spread by lice is also a problem in areas with social unrest and chronic poverty.

How are body lice spread?

Body lice spread through direct physical contact, and through infested clothing, bedding, and towels. This is especially a problem in homeless, transient populations and among groups that have little access to clean clothes and regular bathing facilities.

How are infestations of body lice diagnosed?

Diagnosis is by visual inspection of the seams of clothing and bedding to detect signs of eggs and crawling live lice. Often a magnifying glass is required to make a definitive determination.

Frequently Asked Questions - Pubic Lice

Although it is recommended that you read the entire text regarding pubic lice, the following are some of the most frequently asked questions about the diagnosis, treatment, and eradication of these parasites.

What are pubic lice?

The popular name for pubic lice is "crabs." They are parasitic insects that infest the genital area of humans. The parasites are found around the world and are not tied to a particular race, ethnic group, or social strata.

What do pubic lice look like?

Like all lice, pubic lice have a three-stage life cycle that begins with yellowish white eggs or nits that make 6-10 days to hatch. The immature nymphs begin to feed on blood and mature over a period of 2-3 weeks.

When viewed under magnification, adults have six legs, with the front two being larger and resembling the claws of a crab. They are tan to grayish white.

Where are pubic lice found?

Pubic lice infest the hair in the pubic area and may migrate to coarse hair on the legs, under the arms, in beards and mustaches, or on the eyebrows and eyelashes. If found on the eyebrows or eyelashes of small children, pubic lice are an indicator of sexual abuse.

What are the symptoms of pubic lice?

The most prevalent symptom is intense itching in the genital area. The lice eggs and crawling lice may both be visible, especially under magnification.

How are pubic lice transmitted?

Pubic lice are typically spread through sexual contact in adults. Occasionally transmission my occur from clothing, bedding, or towels. Pubic lice cannot be transmitted from sitting on a toilet seat as the parasites are not equipped to grip smooth surfaces.

How are pubic lice diagnosed?

Typically pubic lice are found when a nit or live louse is seen in the pubic region. Intense itching may actually be the first sign, and a magnified examination by a qualified healthcare provider may be necessary to definitively determine the presence of the parasites.

Once a diagnosis is confirmed, the affected individual should be tested for the presence of any other sexually transmitted diseases.

Frequently Asked Questions - Scabies

Although it is recommended that you read the entire text regarding scabies, the following are some of the most frequently asked questions about the diagnosis, treatment, and eradication of these parasites.

What is scabies?

The human itch mite, a microscopic parasite, burrows into the upper skin layer and lays its eggs. This infestation, characterized by a pimple-like rash and intense itching, is referred to as "scabies" and is spread via skin-to-skin contact.

The condition is present in populations around the world and is not tied to any particular race or social class. Scabies tends to spread most readily in crowded conditions and is especially problematic in nursing homes, extended care facilities, child care facilities, and prisons.

What is crusted or Norwegian scabies?

This more severe form of scabies often affects people with compromised immune systems. The elderly and disabled individuals are at especially high risk.

Due to the very high numbers of mites and eggs present, affected individuals suffer from thick crusts on the skin that are highly contagious. Great care must be taken with clothing, bedding, and furniture to avoid spread of the infestation.

Quick and highly aggressive treatment is required in these cases.

How soon do symptoms of scabies present?

In first instances of scabies infestation, symptoms may not present for 4-6 weeks. The infected person can spread the mites during this time. If a person has had scabies before, the symptoms will appear within 1-4 days of exposure.

What are the symptoms of a scabies infestation?

The two most common symptoms are intense itching at night and a pimple-like rash that may affect most of the body or be localized at the wrist, elbow, armpit, between the fingers, on the nipples, penis, along the waist, or over the buttocks. Tiny blister and scales may be present, and skin sores can develop as a consequence of scratching.

Sometimes tiny burrows are visible on the skin where the female mites are tunneling. The burrows are raised and cooked, and may appear as grayish-white to flesh colored lines.

Because only a few mites may be present, these burrows can be difficult to find as they are often located in folds of skin. In very young children, the head, face, neck, palms, and soles of the feet are often affected.

How is scabies spread?

To be spread, scabies requires prolonged, direct, skin-to-skin contact. Generally a hug or handshake is not sufficient.

Transmission within households and between sexual partners is common. The mites can also travel from person to person on shared clothing, bedding, and towels, but this is more typical in cases of crusted scabies.

How is scabies diagnosed?

Typically the diagnosis of scabies is visual based on the location and appearance of the rash and the distinctive burrows.

The most definitive diagnosis, however, is by identifying the mites themselves, their eggs, or their fecal matter.

Often this is accomplished by removing a mite from the end of a burrow with the tip of a needle or by taking a skin scraping.

How long do the scabies mites live?

Scabies mites can live on a host for 1-2 months, but will not survive for more than 48-72 hours off a human being. When exposed to a temperature of 122 F (50 C), the mites die in 10 minutes.

How is scabies treated?

The products used to treat scabies are called scabicides. Most kill the adult mites, but some are effective against the eggs, but no viable treatment can be obtained over the counter. A prescription for a doctor is required, and all instructions must be followed to the letter.

In adults and older children, the lotion is applied to the entire body, but in young children it is typically used on the head and neck only. It should not be washed off sooner than directed and clean clothes should be worn afterwards.

In households, all members of the family — even if they show no signs of scabies — should be treated at the same time. Re-treatment may be required in 2-4 weeks if itching continues.

Can I get scabies from my pet?

Pets can be infested with a different kind of scabies mite, but they cannot spread the infestation to humans. If a person comes into contact with an infected animal, temporary itching and a skin irritation may occur, but there will be no actual parasitical infestation.

How can I remove scabies mites from my house and clothing?

The scabies mite will not survive off a human host for more than 2-3 days. Wash all items in hot water and dry on the highest setting possible to kill the mites. Anything that cannot be washed or dry cleaned should be sealed in a plastic bag for at least 72 hours. Fumigation is not recommended due to its extreme toxicity and limited effectiveness.

Appendix 1- Lice and Scabies in Animals

Lice do not commonly infest dogs and cats, and pets are not a vector in transferring lice infestations to humans. There is absolutely no reason to subject your pet to any kind of "treatment" if anyone in the house is dealing with a lice problem.

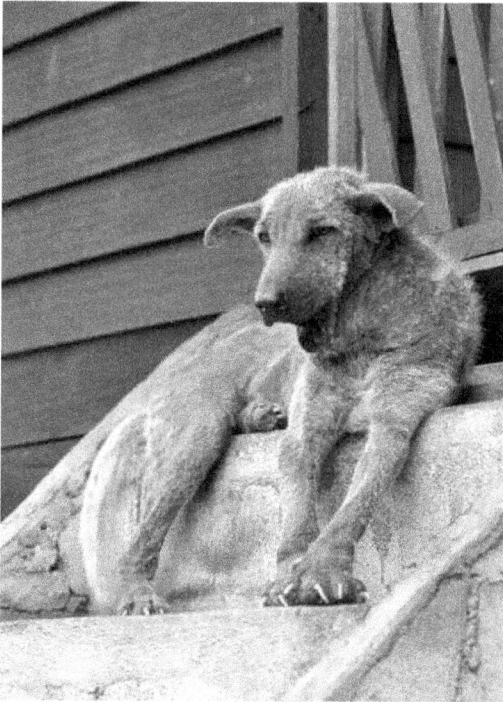

Lice and Pets

Infestations of lice can occur in any animal that has hair, but typically the parasites are only seen on creatures living in crowded, filthy, deplorable conditions.

Appendix 1- Lice and Scabies in Animals

It is important to remember that lice are host specific, meaning that humans get human lice, dogs get dog lice, cats get cat lice, and so forth. Even if a dog louse did get on a human, it wouldn't stay there because the host environment is not correct to facilitate its life cycle.

Dog Lice

There are two types of lice that can infest dogs:

- *Trichodectes canis* is a parasite that chews on the animal's skin.

- *Linognathus setosus* feeds on the dog's blood.

Of the two, *Linognathus setosus* causes the greatest amount of irritation.

Cat Lice

There is only one type of lice that can affect cats, *Felicola subrostrata*. It is a chewing louse, and is seen very rarely.

Symptoms in Dogs and Cats

If dogs or cats are infested with lice, they will scratch incessantly to address the severe itching caused by the parasites.

The coats will become dry and "scruffy" in appearance, often with bald patches and sores present.

Appendix 1- Lice and Scabies in Animals

Typically the lice will be at their greatest concentrations around the ears, neck, and shoulders, with concentrations near and under the tail as well.

(Note that these are the same areas typically infested by fleas.)

Treatment Options

Lice in dogs and cats are treated in much the same fashion as treatment for humans. Insecticide shampoos and powders are used, with a series of re-applications over a 2-3 week period to stay ahead of the parasites' reproductive cycle.

Often if the coat is matted, the vet will recommend shaving your pet. This has the added benefit of making it easier to inspect the skin for the continued presence of live lice.

Wash the animal's bedding in 128.3 F / 53.5 C water and dry on the hottest cycle possible. (Some pet owners prefer to simply discard the bedding. If so, seal the items in plastic bags.)

It is not necessary to use any kind of fogger or fumigant, and in fact, this practice is highly discouraged due to the extreme toxicity of these products.

If the infestation is judged severe, it is imperative that your pet be removed from the area before the fumigant product is used and not be returned until the premises have been thoroughly aired out.

Scabies and Pets

Animals do not spread scabies in humans. Like lice, the mites that cause scabies are species specific. Pets can develop a form of scabies, that is referred to as "mange," but it is not communicable to humans.

Animals with Mange

If a human comes into contact with an animal that has mange, it is possible for the mite to get under the skin and cause temporary itching and irritation.

For this reason, it is important to take precautions when treating a pet with a mange infestation. However, it is equally important to understand that the mites causing the mange cannot live or reproduce on a human host.

The mites from an animal with mange will die on a human within 2 days, and no treatment beyond pallitive ointments to control itching are required.

Treatment Options

Any animal with mange requires the assistance of a qualified veterinarian. As in humans, the condition causes severe itching. The pet will scratch vigorously and wound itself by breaking the skin.

Once this occurs, a viscious circle of hair loss and open sores makes the animal suscptable to secondary fungal and bacterial infections. The resulting stress on the system is quite severe.

There are three types of mites that cause mange in dogs:

- *Cheyletiella*
- *Demodex*
- *Sarcoptes*

Each requires a different treatment protocol, typically comprised of topical medications, dips, and baths.

There are two mites that cause mange in cats:

- *Demodex gatoi*
- *Demodex cati*

In approximately 90% of cases, mange in cats resolves spontaneously, although sulphur dips can speed the process. The animal's overall health condition should be evaluated, however, as mange in cats can be caused by an impaired immune system.

Stray Animals and Mange

In case of stray animals that are malnourished and neglected, mange coupled with weight loss can have fatal consequences.

Appendix 1- Lice and Scabies in Animals

Do not refuse to help a stray animal with mange out of fear that you will contract the condition. If possible, wear gloves, but understand that the creature is in no way to blame for its condition.

Be advised that animal shelters typically will not take strays with mange as the condition is highly communicable in a closed shelter environment.

Appendix II – Available Products

These products and prices represent a small list of items that you can purchase on Amazon US and Amazon UK at the time of publication of this book. I have not personally used these products and cannot vouch for their effectiveness.

USA

Lice Treatments

LiceMD

Regular Kit - $24.86
Pesticide Free Kit -$12.69

Lice R Gone Products (non-toxic)

Lice R Gone® Shampoo (8 oz.) $25.95
Lice R Gone® (1/2 oz. Packet) $5.95
Plastic Nit Comb $0.55
Nano-UV™ Disinfection Scanner $79.95
Nano-UV™ Disinfection Wand $159.95

Licefree Spray, Instant Head Lice Treatment Spray Bottle With Metal Comb, 6-Ounce - $7.21

NitFree Mouse – 4 oz. pump $10.50
NitFree Enzyme Treatment – 16 oz. spray - $15.95
NitFree Enzyme Treatment – 8 oz. spray - $12.95

NitFree Foamer Enzyme Treatment – 8 oz. $15.95

Scabies Treatments

All Stop Scabies & Mite Combo
4 oz. Mitactin Deep Cleaning Salve
8 oz. Mitactin Skin Spray,
2 oz. Mitactin Skin Spray - Travel Size
$39.80

Naturasil Homeopathic Remedies
Topical Cream - 4 oz.
$36.66

Scabies Liquid Soad Treatment
8 oz.
$24.95

Appendix II – Available Products

U.K.

Lice Treatments

Classicure Lice Busting Lotion
200 ml
£5.68

125 ml
£5.59

Professor Melhorn's Picksan Lice Stop Shampoo
100 ml
£6.50

Full Marks Head Lice Soluction with Comb – 4 Treatments
200 ml
£8.00

Hedrin Lotion Head Lice Treatment
150 ml
£8.99

Scabies Treatments

Lyclear Dermal Cream for Scabies and Crab Lice
30 g
£6.25

Appendix II – Available Products

Frequently Used Terms

head lice - Parasitical insects that infest the human scalp and cause intense itching. The condition is properly referred to as pediculosis.

lice - Lice are wingless, flat insects that feed on blood. In humans three types are typically seen: head lice, body lice, and pubic lice.

nymphs - All lice have a three-part life cycle. The second, immature phase of that cycle is the nymph, which matures into adult form in a period of roughly 7-10 days.

Lindane - Lindane is an agricultural pesticide used topically in the treatment of lice and scabies. It has, however, been banned in 52 countries and the state of California and is now used only in extreme resistant cases.

louse - "Louse" is the singular form of the term "lice," a wingless, parasitical insect that infests humans and animals in various forms.

nit - The first stage of the three-phase life cycle seen in lice is the nit or egg.

pediculicide - An treatment agent that is purchased over the counter or prescribed for the express purpose of killing head lice, body lice or pubic lice is called a pediculicide. The three most common agents present in these products are permethrin, pyrethrum, and lindane.

Frequently Used Terms

pediculosis - The proper terms for an infestation of lice present on the human scalp, body or pubic area.

permethrin - This is a topical insecticide that is used to treat various forms of lice and scabies, as well as some species of ticks.

pyrethrum - An insecticide used extensively for the treatment of head lice, nits and scabies.

Scholarly Resources - Lice

For those readers interested in the scholarly literature on lice, the following sampling of articles surveys the period of study from 2000 to 2013.

Abdel-Ghaffar, Fathy, and Semmler, Margit. "Efficacy of Neem Seed Extract Shampoo on Head Lice of Naturally Infected Humans in Egypt." *Parasitology Research* 100, no. 2 (2007): 329-32.

Araújo, Adauto, Ferreira, LF, Guidon, N, Maues da Serra Freire, N, Reinhard, KJ, and Dittmar, K. "Ten Thousand Years of Head Lice Infection." *Parasitology Today* 16, no. 7 (2000): 269.

Canyon, Deon V, Speare, Richard, and Muller, Reinhold. "Spatial and Kinetic Factors for the Transfer of Head Lice (pediculus Capitis) Between Hairs." *Journal of Investigative Dermatology* 119, no. 3 (2002): 629-31.

Downs, AMR, Stafford, KA, Hunt, LP, Ravenscroft, JC, and Coles, GC. "Widespread Insecticide Resistance in Head Lice to the Over-the-Counter Pediculocides in England, and the Emergence of Carbaryl Resistance." *British Journal of Dermatology* 146, no. 1 (2002): 88-93.

Frankowski, Barbara L, and Weiner, Leonard B. "Head Lice." *Pediatrics* 110, no. 3 (2002): 638-43.

Hunter, JA, and Barker, SC. "Susceptibility of Head Lice (pediculus Humanus Capitis) to Pediculicides in Australia." *Parasitology Research* 90, no. 6 (2003): 476-78.

Lee, Si Hyeock, Yoon, Kyong-Sup, Williamson, Martin S, Goodson, Susannah J, Takano-Lee, Miwako, Edman, John D, Devonshire, Alan L, and Marshall Clark, J. "Molecular Analysis of Kdr-like Resistance in Permethrin-resistant Strains of Head Lice, Pediculus Capitis." *Pesticide Biochemistry and Physiology* 66, no. 2 (2000): 130-43.

Leo, NP, Campbell, N J H, Yang, X, Mumcuoglu, K, and Barker, SC. "Evidence From Mitochondrial DNA That Head Lice and Body Lice of Humans (phthiraptera: Pediculidae) Are Conspecific." *Journal of Medical Entomology* 39, no. 4 (2002): 662-66.

Meinking, Terri L, Serrano, Lidia, Hard, Bruce, Entzel, Pamela, Lemard, Glendene, Rivera, Elisabeth, and Villar, Maria Elena. "Comparative in Vitro Pediculicidal Efficacy of Treatments in a Resistant Head Lice Population in the United States." *Archives of Dermatology* 138, no. 2 (2002): 220.

Pearlman, Dale Lawrence. "A Simple Treatment for Head Lice: Dry-on, Suffocation-based Pediculicide." *Pediatrics* 114, no. 3 (2004): e275-79.

Reed, David L, Smith, Vincent S, Hammond, Shaless L, Rogers, Alan R, and Clayton, Dale H. "Genetic Analysis of Lice Supports Direct Contact Between Modern and Archaic Humans." *PLoS biology* 2, no. 11 (2004): e340.

Roberts, Richard J. "Head Lice." *New England Journal of Medicine* 346, no. 21 (2002): 1645-50.

Roberts, RJ, Casey, D, Morgan, DA, and Petrovic, M. "Comparison of Wet Combing With Malathion for Treatment of Head Lice in the Uk: a Pragmatic Randomised Controlled Trial." *The Lancet* 356, no. 9229 (2000): 540-44.

Sasaki, Toshinori, Kobayashi, Mutsuo, and Agui, Noriaki. "Detection of Bartonella Quintana From Body Lice (anoplura: Pediculidae) Infesting Homeless People in Tokyo By Molecular Technique." *Journal of Medical Entomology* 39, no. 3 (2002): 427-29.

Sim, Seobo, Lee, In-Yong, Lee, Kyu-Jae, Seo, Jang-Hoon, Im, Kyung-Il, Shin, Myeong Heon, and Yong, Tai-Soon. "A Survey on Head Lice Infestation in Korea (2001) and the Therapeutic Efficacy of Oral Trimethoprim/sulfamethoxazole Adding to Lindane Shampoo." *The Korean Journal of Parasitology* 41, no. 1 (2003): 57-61.

Willems, Sara, Lapeere, Hilde, Haedens, Nele, Pasteels, Inge, Naeyaert, Jean-Marie, and De Maeseneer, Jan. "The Importance of Socio-economic Status and Individual Characteristics on the Prevalence of Head Lice in Schoolchildren." *European Journal of Dermatology* 15, no. 5 (2005): 387-92.

Scholarly Resources – Scabies

For those readers interested in the scholarly literature on scabies, the following sampling of articles surveys the period of study from 2000 to 2013.

Andriantsoanirina, V, Izri, A, Botterel, F, Foulet, F, Chosidow, O, and Durand, R. "Molecular Survey of Knockdown Resistance to Pyrethroids in Human Scabies Mites." *Clin Microbiol Infect* (2013).

Antonucci, VA, Balestri, R, Sgubbi, P, Magnano, M, Tengattini, V, and Bardazzi, F. "Atypical Presentation of Scabies: a Single Nodule of the Scalp in a Child." *G Ital Dermatol Venereol* 148, no. 5 (2013): 546-47.

Banzhaf, CA, Themstrup, L, Ring, HC, Welzel, J, Mogensen, M, and Jemec, GB. "In Vivo Imaging of Sarcoptes Scabiei Infestation Using Optical Coherence Tomography." *Case Rep Dermatol* 5, no. 2 (2013): 156-62.

Barreiros, H, Alves, J, and Serrano, P. "[norwegian Scabies]." *Acta Med Port* 26, no. 3 (2013): 287.

Bernard, J, Depaepe, L, and Balme, B. "[histopathology of Scabies.]." *Ann Dermatol Venereol* 140, no. 10 (2013): 656-57.

Boureau, AS, Cozic, C, Poiraud, C, Varin, S, Chaillous, B, and Cormier, G. "Does Immunodepression Induced By Tnf Antagonists Promote Atypical Scabies?" *Joint Bone Spine* (2013):

Davis, JS, McGloughlin, S, Tong, SY, Walton, SF, and Currie, BJ. "A Novel Clinical Grading Scale to Guide the Management of Crusted Scabies." *PLoS Negl Trop Dis* 7, no. 9 (2013): e2387.

Elston, CA, and Elston, DM. "Treatment of Common Skin Infections and Infestations During Pregnancy." *Dermatol Ther* 26, no. 4 (2013): 312-20.

Engelman, D, Kiang, K, Chosidow, O, McCarthy, J, Fuller, C, Lammie, P, Hay, R, Steer, A, On, Behalf Of The Members Of The International Alliance For The Control Of Scabies, and Iacs. "Toward the Global Control of Human Scabies: Introducing the International Alliance for the Control of Scabies." *PLoS Negl Trop Dis* 7, no. 8 (2013): e2167.

Goldust, M, and Rezaee, E. "Comparative Trial of Oral Ivermectin Versus Sulfur 8% Ointment for the Treatment of Scabies." *J Cutan Med Surg* 17, no. 5 (2013): 299-300.

Goldust, M, Rezaee, E, Raghifar, R, and Naghavi-Behzad, M. "Comparison of Permethrin 2.5 % Cream Vs. Tenutex Emulsion for the Treatment of Scabies." *Ann Parasitol* 59, no. 1 (2013): 31-35.

Goldust, M, Rezaee, E, Raghifar, R, and Naghavi-Behzad, M. "Ivermectin Vs. Lindane in the Treatment of Scabies." *Ann Parasitol* 59, no. 1 (2013): 37-41.

Govindarajan, R, Mitra, S, Obiechina, N, and Weeraman, S. "Norwegian Scabies." *Br J Hosp Med (Lond)* 74, no. 8 (2013): 471-Unknown.

Gray, S, Lennon, D, Anderson, P, Stewart, J, and Farrell, E. "Nurse-led School-based Clinics for Skin Infections and Rheumatic Fever Prevention: Results From a Pilot Study in South Auckland." *N Z Med J* 126, no. 1373 (2013): 53-61.

Hossain, D. "Using Methotrexate to Treat Patients With Enl Unresponsive to Steroids and Clofazimine: a Report on 9 Patients." *Lepr Rev* 84, no. 1 (2013): 105-12.

Ito, T. "Mazzotti Reaction With Eosinophilia After Undergoing Oral Ivermectin for Scabies." *J Dermatol* 40(9), no. 9 (2013): 776-77.

McLean, FE. "The Elimination of Scabies: a Task for Our Generation." *Int J Dermatol* 52, no. 10 (2013): 1215-23.

Mohebbipour, A, Saleh, P, Goldust, M, Amirnia, M, Zadeh, YJ, Mohamad, RM, and Rezaee, E. "Comparison of Oral Ivermectin Vs. Lindane Lotion 1% for the Treatment of Scabies." *Clin Exp Dermatol* 38, no. 7 (2013): 719-23.

Morgan, MS, Arlian, LG, and Markey, MP. "Sarcoptes Scabiei Mites Modulate Gene Expression in Human Skin Equivalents." *PLoS One* 8, no. 8 (2013): e71143.

Shimose, L, and Munoz-Price, LS. "Diagnosis, Prevention, and Treatment of Scabies." *Curr Infect Dis Rep* 15, no. 5 (2013): 426-31.

Thapa, DP, Jha, AK, Kharel, C, and Shrestha, S. "Dermatological Problems in Geriatric Patients: a Hospital Based Study." *Nepal Med Coll J* 14, no. 3 (2012): 193-95.

Tidman, AS, and Tidman, MJ. "Intense Nocturnal Itching Should Raise Suspicion of Scabies." *Practitioner* 257, no. 1761 (2013): 23-7, 2.

Tucker, R, Patel, M, Layton, AL, and Walton, S. "An Exploratory Study Demonstrating the Diagnostic Ability of Healthcare Professionals in Primary Care Using Online Case Studies for Common Skin Conditions." *Int J Pharm Pract* (2013):

Index

www.ingramcontent.com/pod-product-compliance
Lightning Source LLC
Chambersburg PA
CBHW072237290326
41934CB00008BB/1325